Lose weight in 14 days with low carb high protein diet

Table of Contents

Introduction

I want to thank you and congratulate you for downloading the book, *"Low Carb: Low Carb, High Protein Diet Plan With Delicious Recipes - Ultimate 14 Days To Rapid Weight Loss, Belly Fat Reduction (Cookbook To Achieve Lean Muscles And Healthy Life)."*

We have been told growing up that carbohydrates are the body's main source of energy and owing to these; over time, we have increased our carbohydrate intake because of the great importance placed on carbohydrates.

However, while carbohydrates are great, the greatest problem is that our diet is too high in carbohydrates. The average person takes a cup of tea or coffee with bread, muffin, or pancake or a bowl of cereal with milk. They then take rice or pasta for lunch, an afternoon snack high in carbohydrates like cookies and in the evening, they eat rice or pasta and a high carbohydrate dessert.

This is clearly too much carbohydrate than your body actually needs. Thus, the body will break down the carbohydrates into glucose and use glucose for energy with the excess being converted to fat and stored. The stored fat is for use during starvation or periods when your body cannot get glucose. However, starvation is not something that many Americans have to deal with so the extra fat is not used and as you continue to eat more carbohydrates; your body continues accumulating more fat. Before you know it, you are overweight or obese and plagued with a number of diseases like diabetes.

If you want to lose weight, feel great, and build muscle, you have to do something about the situation; you need to manage your carbohydrate intake. This is where a low carb diet comes in. This diet is low in carb, high in protein and fat and is very effective for weight loss.

This book will explain a low carb diet better to help you understand what it is, how it works, how it is beneficial, and a 14-week meal plan to help you get started with the diet.

Thanks again for downloading this book. I hope you enjoy it!

Low Carb Diet Defined

A low carb diet is simply a diet that limits the consumption of carbs. For instance, foods high in carbohydrates like bread, pastas, and sugary foods. However, carbohydrates are also found in other foods such as beans, vegetables, and milk.

Adopting a low carb diet has been known to be quite effective at weight loss. This is because the current American diet is too high in carbohydrates, which means that once your body breaks down the carbohydrates into glucose, it uses some of it for its functions with the rest being converted to fat and stored. Since we rarely use the stored fat for energy because we are constantly eating excess carbohydrates and not exercising as much, in no time we have gained weight.

With a low carb diet, you reduce your excess carb intake and focus on eating healthy fats and protein, which ensures that you don't store any excess glucose as fat and with the low carb intake, your body will actually start to burn the fat for energy, which leads to weight loss. In addition, fats and protein are more filling; thus, you are likely to eat less and this will definitely lead to weight loss. If you combine a low carb diet with exercise, you will definitely gain lean muscles.

Before moving on to the foods you can eat while on a low carb diet, it is important to know how many grams of carbohydrates per day will help you achieve your weight loss goal. Your daily total carbohydrate intake should be less than 100grams net carbs and in some cases less than 50grams net carbs if you want to lose weight fast.

Net carbs = carbohydrates-fiber

With the restriction of carbs, a low carb diet entails high consumption of proteins and healthy fats to compensate for the low intake of carbohydrates. Let us look at the foods you can eat while on a low carb diet:

Meat - Beef, chicken, pork, lamb and other meats; always go for grass fed.

High fat dairy - Cheese, yogurt, heavy cream, butter

Eggs - all types of eggs are allowed but pastured eggs or Omega-3 enriched eggs are the best.

Fish and seafood - such as Salmon, trout, haddock, and halibut; wild caught fish are the best.

Healthy fats and oils – such as coconut oil, cod fish liver oil, lard, olive oil, and butter.

Vegetables – opt for leafy green vegetables like kale, spinach, cauliflower, broccoli among others.

Nuts and seeds- Walnuts, almonds, sunflower seeds, pumpkin seeds etc.

Fruits - opt for fruits low in fructose like berries, avocado etc.

Please note that all of the foods that you should eat should be unprocessed.

If you exercise frequently, you will need your energy; thus, you can eat the below foods.

Non-gluten grains - Rice, quinoa, oats and any others

Tubers - such as sweet potatoes, potatoes, yams

Legumes - Lentils, pinto beans, black beans etc.

Eat the below foods in moderation

Dark Chocolate - Choose the organic brands that have 70% cocoa or higher.

Wine - it should be dry with no added carbs or sugars

Generally, you should avoid starchy foods such as pasta and wheat as well as processed foods.

Also avoid eating foods high in sugar such as fruit juices, candy, soft drinks and the likes, Trans fats both partly hydrogenated and hydrogenated oils, vegetable oils and high omega 6 seed oils, artificial sweeteners, 'low fat and diet' products and foods that are highly processed.

Let us now get started on the 14 week plan to help you lose weight, gain muscle and look great.

Meal Plan For Week 1

Day 1

Breakfast

Hazelnut Waffles

Servings: 6

Ingredients

1 cup Hazelnut meal

3 tablespoons hazelnut oil

½ teaspoon hazelnut extract

2 tablespoons coconut flour

1/3 cup full-fat Greek yogurt

¼ teaspoons stevia extract

3 tablespoons Swerve Sweetener or granulated erythritol

½ cup Chocolate protein powder

4 large eggs

2 tablespoons cocoa powder

1. Preheat your waffle iron to medium high and your oven to 200 degrees F.

2. Place a wire rack onto a baking sheet.

3. Whisk together the protein powder, hazelnut meal, coconut flour, sweetener and cocoa powder in a large bowl.

4. Add in the hazelnut oil, eggs, stevia, yogurt, hazelnut extract and mix together until well combined.

5. Grease the waffle iron and pour about ¼ to 1/3 of the batter into each part of the iron. Cover up with the lid and let it cook until crisp and browned.

6. Remove gently from the iron when done and place onto prepared baking sheet in the oven to keep warm.

7. Repeat this procedure with the remaining batter. Once done top the waffles with butter, chopped hazelnuts, whipped cream, sugar-free syrup, berries and whatever else you desire. Enjoy!

Nutritional info: 257 calories, 7g net carbs, 16g protein, 19g fat

Lunch
Chicken Salad with Basil-Lemon Vinaigrette

Servings: 4

Ingredients

Chicken

3 garlic cloves- minced

¾ teaspoon fine grain sea salt

½ teaspoon ground cumin

2 tablespoons lemon juice

¼ teaspoon ground coriander

1 teaspoon curry powder

2 tablespoons olive oil

1 pound free range organic chicken breast- cut it into 3 inch strips

Salad

1 avocado- sliced

1 cup cherry tomatoes- halved

2 handfuls of torn fresh basil leaves

6 cups spring greens

Basil-Lemon Vinaigrette

1 clove garlic- smashed

2 large handfuls fresh basil leaves

½ teaspoon fine grain sea salt

5 tablespoons of olive oil

2 tablespoons fresh lemon juice

Instructions

1. To cook the chicken, whisk together the lemon juice, curry powder, coriander, olive oil, salt, garlic, and cumin in a bowl until well combined.

2. Put the chicken strips in a Ziploc bag or a sealable container, pour in the marinade, and combine.

3. Seal or cover and place in the refrigerator for about 20 minutes to marinate (you can marinate overnight to get the best flavor).

4. Once you are ready to make the meal, place a large non-stick skillet over medium high heat.

5. Add in a bit of olive oil together with the chicken and cook as you turn regularly until the chicken is cooked through and golden brown. This will take about 6- 8 minutes.

6. Meanwhile, make the vinaigrette. Use a small blender or a food processor to combine the garlic, lemon juice, basil, and salt until smooth. As the motor is running, add in the oil slowly and keep on blending until combined; set aside.

7. To make the salad, put the greens in a bowl and toss them with a dash of pepper and salt. Place the chicken on top together with the avocado, basil and tomatoes. Drizzle the lemon basil vinaigrette all over the bowl of salad and serve!

Nutritional info: 392 calories, 27g protein, 9g carbs, 28g fat

Dinner

Grilled Salmon Kebobs

Servings: 4

Ingredients

Salmon

1 pound of salmon- without skin and cut into around 12 cubes

Marinade

2 cloves garlic- minced

2 tablespoons lemon juice

3 tablespoons minced fresh rosemary

2 tablespoons extra virgin olive oil

½ teaspoon kosher or sea salt

1 tablespoon Dijon mustard

½ teaspoon black pepper

4 skewers, if you use bamboo or wood soak in warm water for 20-30 minutes

Instructions

1. Mix all the marinade ingredients in a bowl.

2. Add in the salmon and allow it to marinate for at least 20 minutes at room temperature.

3. Thread in the cubes of salmon onto the skewers.

4. Coat a grill pan, skillet or grates of grill using a light layer of cooking spray and set to high.

5. Once it is hot, place the skewers onto the grill or pan and let them cook for three minutes on each side until the fish flakes easily with a fork and is opaque.

6. Baste with any marinade that is leftover as you cook. Serve the kebabs with steamed broccoli.

Nutritional info: 308 calories, 24g protein, 1g net carbs, 22g fat

Day 2

Breakfast
Hazelnut waffles

Lunch
Grilled Halloumi Salad

Servings: 1

Ingredients

0.5 ounces chopped walnuts

5 grape tomatoes

Balsamic vinegar

Salt

1 handful baby arugula

Olive oil

1 Persian cucumber

3 ounces Halloumi cheese

Instructions

1. Cut the cheese into 1/3 inch slices. Don't make them too thin because when put on the grill, they will shrink a little.

2. Place the Halloumi cheese on the grill and grill for 3 to 5 minutes on each side after which you will see nice grill marks on the sides.

3. Prepare the salad by first washing then cutting the veggies. Cut the tomatoes in half and the cucumber into small slices. Add the tomatoes and cucumbers to a bowl. Add in the walnuts and baby arugula.

4. When the cheese has the grill marks on each side, place on top of the salad and sprinkle some salt on top. Dress with balsamic vinegar and olive oil then serve!

Nutritional info: 560 calories, 47g fat, 21g protein, 7g carbs

Dinner
Zucchini Noodle Carbonara

Servings: 4

Ingredients

4 slices (nitrate-free) Canadian bacon/ deli ham - diced

½ teaspoon fresh ground black pepper

2 egg yolks

¼ cup grated Parmesan cheese

1 egg

½ teaspoon sea salt

4 large zucchini

Instructions

1. Use a julienne peeler or a spiral slicer to cut the zucchini into noodles.

2. Lay the prepared noodles on a paper towel and sprinkle some salt evenly on top.

3. Allow the zucchini noodles to rest for about 5 minutes then squeeze out as much liquid as possible.

4. Whisk together the cheese, egg and egg yolk until well combined.

5. Place a skillet over medium heat and add in the bacon. Cook until crisp.

6. Add in the zucchini noodles and stir until they are warmed through.

7. Lower the heat and add in the egg mixture. Turn off the heat then stir the noodles until the eggs are just about cooked.

8. Season with some black pepper just before you serve!

Nutritional info: 308calories, 16g fat, 12g net carbs, 28g protein

Day 3

Breakfast
Spinach Enchilada Omelet

Servings: 6

Ingredients

1 teaspoon olive oil

1 medium avocado- diced

Salt and pepper- to taste

½ cup of scallions- chopped (and more for garnish)

3 cups egg whites or egg whites from 18 large eggs

1 medium ripe tomato- diced

1 cup green enchilada sauce

2 tablespoons cilantro- chopped

10 ounces package frozen spinach

4.5 ounces can of chopped green chiles

Kosher salt and fresh ground pepper

2 tablespoons water

Cooking spray

1 ½ cups grated colby-jack cheese

1. At the bottom of a 9 x 12 inch baking sheet pour in 1/3 cup of enchilada sauce and preheat your oven to 350 degrees F.

2. Whisk together the water, egg whites, and a pinch of pepper and salt.

3. Use cooking spray to lightly coat a large non-stick skillet and place it over medium heat.

4. Add in ¼ of the egg whites (1/2 a cup) and swirl to cover the bottom of the pan evenly. Cook for about 2 minutes until set. Flip the egg over and cook it for one more minute until set. Place aside on a dish and repeat with the rest of the eggs until all the egg tortillas (approximately 6) are cooked and set aside.

5. Place a nonstick skillet over medium heat and add in oil to heat. Add in the scallions and cook for about 2 to 3 minutes until fragrant (but not browned). Add in the cilantro and tomato and season with salt as desired and cook for a minute more until soft.

6. Stir in the green chile and spinach and cook for 5 more minutes (adjust the pepper and salt as desired).

7. Remove from the heat and add in ½ cup of the Colby Jack cheese. Mix well to combine.

8. Divide the spinach among the egg tortillas (about 1/3 cup each) and roll them up. Place them with the seam side down in a baking dish. Top with the rest of the enchilada sauce and the cheese that remained and cover with foil.

9. Bake until the cheese is melted and the tortillas are hot; for about 20- 25 minutes.

10. Serve with scallions and diced avocado.

Nutritional info: 239 calories, 12g fat, 6g net carbs, 24g protein

Lunch
Zucchini shrimp scampi

Servings: 4

Ingredients

¼ cup chicken stock

Kosher salt and freshly ground black pepper, to taste

3 cloves garlic- minced

½ teaspoon red pepper flakes, or more to taste

4 medium-sized zucchini- spiralized

1 pound medium shrimp- peeled and deveined

2 tablespoons chopped parsley

Juice of 1 lemon

2 tablespoons freshly grated Parmesan cheese

2 tablespoons unsalted butter

Instructions

1. Add the butter to a large skillet and heat it over medium high heat.

2. Add in the red pepper flakes, shrimp, and garlic and cook as you stir occasionally for about 2 to 3 minutes or until pink.

3. Stir in the lemon juice and the chicken stock and season with pepper and salt as desired.

4. Bring the mixture to a simmer and stir in the zucchini noodles for about 1 to 2 minutes until they are well incorporated.

5. Serve right away with parsley and parmesan if desired and enjoy!

Nutritional info: 214.3 calories, 5.9g net carbs, 27g protein, 8.6g fat

Dinner
Slow cooker lemon garlic chicken

Servings: 4

Ingredients

3 tablespoons lemon juice

½ teaspoon oregano

¾ cup chicken broth

2 tablespoons garlic- minced

1 lemon- sliced

2 pounds of chicken breast

¼ teaspoon pepper

½ teaspoon salt

½ teaspoon garlic powder

1 teaspoon basil

Instructions

1. Mix all the seasonings in a small medium bowl and rub this seasoning on all sides of the chicken breasts.

2. Grease a skillet over medium heat and add the chicken. Brown it on both sides for 7 to 10 minutes.

3. Add each of the cooked chicken breast to a slow cooker. Place a slice of lemon on each breast and put all the remaining slices under or in between the chicken.

4. Pour the chicken broth into the slow cooker over the chicken. Cover then cook it on high for 3 to 4 hours or on low for 6 to 7 hours. Serve when ready with some vegetables.

Nutritional info: 65 calories, 1.75g net carbs, 9g protein, 1.4g fat

Day 4

Breakfast
Cheesy eggs

Servings: 4

Ingredients

¼ cup chives- chopped

4 eggs

Pepper to taste

¼ cup Parmesan cheese-shredded

3 strips cooked bacon- crumbled

Instructions

1. Separate the egg yolks from the egg whites and put the whites in a large metal bowl and the yolks in 4 separate bowls or in the broken egg shells.

2. Whip the whites in a metal mixing bowl until still peaks are formed. Fold in the bacon, cheese, and chives carefully.

3. Use parchment paper to line a baking sheet and spoon four mounds of the whipped egg whites onto it. Make a deep hole at the center of each mound using the back of a spoon.

4. Bake for 3 minutes at 450 degrees then remove from the oven.

5. Place a yolk in each hole and sprinkle some pepper on top to taste.

6. Put back into the oven and bake for about 2 to 3 minutes to have a soft egg yolk. Serve right away and enjoy!

Nutritional info: 161 calories, 13.7g protein, 1.1g carbs, 11.4g fats

Lunch
Previous night's dinner

Dinner
Grilled Salmon Kebabs

Day 5

Breakfast
Cheesy Eggs

Lunch
Tangy Chicken Salad

Servings: 1

Ingredients

3-ounce boneless skinless chicken breast

1 cup spring mix

1 tablespoon chopped onion

1 cup romaine lettuce

1 tablespoon dried cranberries

2 tablespoons red pepper dressing

½ cup mandarin oranges

1 teaspoon sunflower seed kernels

Salt, pepper, and garlic powder to taste

Instructions

1. Dry the chicken and season it on both sides.

2. Pan sear or grill the chicken until it is cooked through (an internal temp of 165 degrees F).

3. Allow the chicken to rest for at least 3 minutes on top of a cutting board and then slice it against the grain.

4. Toss everything in a bowl and drizzle some dressing on top.

Nutritional info: 286 calories, 10.5g fat, 18g net carbs, 27.1g protein

Dinner
Tasty Meatballs

Servings: 4 (5 meatballs each)

Ingredients

Salt and pepper to taste

1 pound ground beef

2 cups reduced sodium beef stock

½ teaspoon allspice

1 clove garlic- minced

2 ounces light cream cheese

1 large egg

¼ cup seasoned breadcrumbs

¼ cup minced parsley

1 teaspoon olive oil

1 small onion- minced

1 celery stalk- minced

Instructions

1. Heat the oil in a large deep pan over medium heat.

2. Toss in the onions and garlic, and sauté for about 4 to 5 minutes until the onions are translucent. Add in the parsley and celery and cook for 3 to 4 more minutes until soft. Allow it cool for a few minutes.

3. Combine the egg, breadcrumbs, pepper, beef, onion mixture, salt and allspice and mix well.

4. Use your hands to form the meatballs, about 1/8 a cup each (you can fill ¼ cup then divide the meat into 2). Put the beef stock into the pan and bring it to a boil. Lower the heat to medium low and add the meatballs gently into the broth. Cover then cook for at least 20 minutes.

5. Remove the meatballs using a slotted spoon and place them in a serving dish.

6. Strain the stock and add to a blender together with the cream cheese and pulse until smooth.

7. Add back to the pan and let it simmer for a few minutes until thick.

8. Serve zucchini noodles with the meatballs and then pour the sauce over the meatballs.

9. Garnish with some parsley and serve.

Nutritional info: 213.5 calories, 10g fat, 25.1g protein, 7.5g net carbs

Day 6

Breakfast

Broccoli Omelet

Servings: 1

Ingredients

1 slice Swiss cheese

½ cup broccoli- cooked

1 tablespoon milk

Salt and fresh pepper

2 egg whites

Oil spray

1 egg

Instructions

1. Beat the egg whites, egg, pepper, salt, and milk in a small bowl.

2. Heat a non-stick skillet over medium heat and spray the pan with oil lightly.

3. Add the eggs when the skillet is warm and rotate the pan to completely cover it with egg. Reduce the heat to low.

4. Lay the cheese in the center of the eggs and top it with broccoli. Once the eggs are set, flip the sides over towards the center to form your omelet.

Nutritional info: 183.2 calories, 20.6g protein, 3.8g net carbs, 8.5g fat

Lunch

Cheeseburger Salad

Servings: 6

Ingredients

¾ cup ranch dressing

Salad

24 cups of romaine lettuce (4 cups for each salad)

3 cups tomatoes- chopped

¾ cup reduced-fat cheddar cheese

Burger Crumble

3 tablespoons Worcestershire sauce

½ teaspoon sea salt

1 pound ground beef

Freshly ground pepper- to taste

1 cup yellow onion- diced

Instructions

1. For the burger crumble: Add the ground beef to a nonstick pan together with the onions and brown for 5 minutes over medium high heat.

2. Cook as you stir to break up the beef into a crumble.

3. Once the beef is browned, transfer the beef to a colander in the sink to drain any fat.

4. Add the beef back to the pan and stir in Worcestershire sauce, pepper, and salt. Reduce the heat to low flame and let it simmer for 5 minutes as you stir often.

5. To make single salad: Line a single dinner plate with 4 cups of lettuce. Top the lettuce with ½ cup of warm burger crumble and sprinkle ½ cup of drained tomatoes. Drizzle 2 tablespoons of the ranch dressing over the salad. Add 2 tablespoons of cheese on top.

6. Pack the burger crumble in different containers and put in the freezer to make more burger salad.

Nutritional info: 242 calories, 9g fat, 15g net carbs, 25g protein

Dinner
Leftovers from lunch

Day 7

Breakfast
Spinach Enchilada omelet

Lunch
Tangy Chicken Salad

Dinner
Tuna-Stuffed Tomatoes

Servings: 4

Ingredients

Salt and pepper

2 tablespoons minced fresh parsley

1 tablespoon capers, drained, rinsed

8 small tomatoes

10 pitted kalamata olives, minced

1 tablespoon olive oil

½ teaspoon minced fresh thyme leaves

2 3 ounces cans oil-packed tuna, drained

Instructions

1. Use paper towels to line a baking sheet then cut a thin slice from the top of each tomato.

2. Scoop out the seeds and the pulp from the tomato leaving the shell intact. Set the shells with the cut side down to drain them on the paper towels.

3. Mix the olives, capers, pepper, parsley, tuna, thyme, and olive oil and break up any large chunks.

4. Season the mixture with some additional pepper and salt if desired. Spoon this mixture into the tomato shells and serve.

Nutritional info: 169 calories, 10g fat, 13g protein, 6g net carbs

Meal Plan For Week 2

Day 1

Breakfast
Microwave-bread

Servings: 1

Ingredients

¼ teaspoon baking powder

1 large egg

1 tablespoon salted butter, melted and slightly cooled

1 tablespoon coconut flour

Instructions

1. Use a fork to mix the ingredients until very smooth.

2. Use a spatula to transfer the mixture to a small Pyrex bowl and microwave it on high for 90 seconds.

3. The bread will puff up as you 'bake' then it will deflate. It will look like a muffin when done and if it is not set cook in the microwave for 30 more seconds but don't overcook it as it will dry up.

4. Use a small knife to gently loosen the bread edges and remove the bread from the bowl to a plate. Slice it into 2 and top it with your favorite toppings. Enjoy with a cup of coffee or tea!

Nutritional info: 204.6 calories, 2.7g net carbs, 17.1g fat, 7.4g protein

Lunch

Salmon with Avocado Tzatziki

Servings: 4

Ingredients

24 ounces salmon, cut into 4 portions

2 tablespoons olive oil

1 teaspoon lemon zest

2 tablespoons lemon juice

1 tablespoon yogurt

1 clove garlic, grated

1 teaspoon oregano

¼ teaspoon salt

¼ teaspoon pepper

2 cups avocado Tzatziki

Tzatziki

1 ripe avocado, mashed

2 tablespoons lemon juice

1 tablespoon fresh dill, chopped

1 clove garlic, grated

½ cup cucumber, peeled, seeded, grated and squeezed to drain

½ plain Greek yogurt

Salt and pepper to taste

Instructions

1. Marinate the salmon in lemon juice, oil, yogurt, zest, oregano, garlic, pepper and salt for about 20 minutes before you place it on baking dish.

2. Bake it in a preheated oven at 400 degrees F or 200 degrees C for about ten minutes until the salmon just starts to flake easily.

3. In the meantime, prepare the avocado tzatziki; mix all the tzatziki ingredients.

4. Once the salmon is ready, serve with the avocado tzatziki.

Nutritional info: 373 calories, 5.7g net carbs, 22.2g fat, 36g protein

Dinner
Grilled Salmon Kebobs

Day 2

Breakfast

Toasted Coconut Cereal

Servings: 4

Ingredients

2 tablespoons of cinnamon

3 ½ cups unsweetened coconut flakes (about 3 ½ cups)

4 tablespoons of granular sweetener (for low carb use Swerve)

2 tablespoons of grass fed butter or ghee

Instructions

1. Preheat your oven to 350 degrees F and put the coconut flakes in a large bowl.

2. Combine the butter, sweetener, and cinnamon in a saucepan over medium heat and heat until they combine perfectly.

3. Pour the sauce all over the coconut and stir it to coat.

4. Spread the coconut over rimmed baking sheet and bake for 5 to 8 minutes as you flip and stir every few minutes to make sure they don't burn.

5. Let it cool and serve with some coconut milk or almond milk.

Nutritional info: 7.87 g net carbs (add carbs count for the sweetener you use)

Lunch

Pecan crusted chicken

Servings: 7

Ingredients

1 pound boneless, skinless chicken breast tenders

1 teaspoon salt

3 teaspoons water

2 eggs

½ teaspoon garlic powder

1 cup almond flour

¼ teaspoon cayenne pepper

1 cup chopped pecan pieces

½ teaspoon pepper

Instructions

1. Preheat your oven to 375 degrees and use aluminum to line a large baking sheet.

2. Crush and mix the pecan pieces, pepper, salt, garlic powder, cayenne powder and almond flour making sure that the pecans are well mixed with all the other ingredients (the pecans should also be finely chopped).

3. Whisk together the water and the eggs in a shallow bowl and place it near the pecan mixture.

4. Dip the chicken in the pecan mixture and shake off the excess. Immerse the chicken into the egg mixture then in the pecan mixture.

5. Ensure that the chicken is covered completely with the pecan mixture.

6. Place the coated chicken on baking sheets and spray both sides with cooking spray ensuring that you don't drench them.

7. Bake until golden brown for 16 to 18 minutes (rotate you pan half way through the mark).

Nutritional info: 181.43 calories, 16.57g protein, 2.43g net carbs

Dinner
Lasagna Stuffed Mushrooms

Servings: 4

Ingredients
3 cloves chopped garlic

2 loose cups baby spinach- chopped

1/3 cup chopped onion

1 teaspoon olive oil
½ cup marinara sauce

Kosher salt

¾ cup part skim ricotta

½ cup grated parmesan cheese

½ cup part skim shredded mozzarella

4 large basil leaves, chopped

1 large egg

1/3 cup chopped red bell pepper

4 large portobella mushroom caps

Instructions

1. Preheat your oven to 400 degrees F and use oil to spray a baking sheet.

2. Remove the stems gently from the mushrooms and take out the gills then spray the tops of the mushrooms with oil and season with fresh pepper and 1/8 teaspoon of salt.

3. Place a large non-stick sauté pan over medium heat and when hot add some oil, red pepper, garlic and onion and add 1/8 teaspoon of salt.

4. Cook for 3 to 4 minutes until soft. Add in the baby spinach and sauté for about a minute until wilted.

5. Add the egg, ricotta and parmesan cheese to a medium bowl and mix well. Add in the basil and the cooked veggies and mix.

6. Use this ricotta mixture to stuff the mushrooms and top them with 2 tablespoons of mozzarella and 2 tablespoons of marinara each.

7. Put in the oven and bake for about 20 to 25 minutes. Garnish with some basil and serve.

Nutritional info: 236 calories, 13g fat, 11.5g net carb, 20g protein

Day 3

Breakfast
Spinach Enchilada Omelet

Lunch
Previous night's dinner

Dinner
Turkey and sweet potato chili

Servings: 5

Ingredients

1 medium sweet potato- peeled then diced into ½ -inch cubes

½ teaspoon cumin, or to taste

Kosher salt to taste

20 ounces ground turkey

10 ounces can tomatoes with green chilies

3 cloves garlic- crushed

½ cup onion- chopped

¼ teaspoon chili powder

¼ teaspoon paprika

1 bay leaf

¾ cup water

8 ounces can tomato sauce

Fresh cilantro- for garnish

Instructions

1. Brown the turkey over medium high heat and break up the chunks as it cooks into smaller pieces then season with cumin and salt.

2. Once the turkey is browned and cooked, add in garlic and onions and cook for about three minutes over medium heat.

3. Add the can of tomatoes, tomato sauce, sweet potato, cumin, paprika, chili, water, bay leaf and salt.

4. Cover and let it simmer, as you stir frequently, for 25 minutes over medium low heat or until the potatoes are cooked through.

5. Add in a ¼ cup of additional water if required; take out the bay leaf, then serve.

Nutritional info: 235 calories, 8g fat, 12g net carbs, 23g protein

Day 4

Breakfast
Toasted Coconut Cereal

Lunch
Cheeseburger Salad

Dinner
Lemon Fish Fillet

Servings: 4

Ingredients

4 (4- 6 ounces) halibut, cod or flounder

2 lemons- one cut in halves, one cut in wedges

3 tablespoons olive oil- divided

¼ teaspoon freshly ground black pepper

¼ teaspoon sea salt

Instructions

1. Let the fish rest in a bowl for 10 to 15 minutes at room temperature.

2. Rub one tablespoon of olive oil and sprinkle some pepper and salt on each side of the fillet.

3. Place a sauté pan or a large skillet over medium heat and add in 2 tablespoons of olive oil.

4. Once the oil is hot and shimmering (not smoking though) add in the fish. Let it cook for about 2 to 3 minutes on each side such that each side is cooked through and browned.

5. Squeeze the lemon halves (both of them) over the fish and then remove the fish from the heat.

6. If some lemon juice is left on the pan pour it on top of the fish as you serve. Serve the fish with lemon wedges.

7. For a full meal: toss some baby kale, arugula (or other lettuce) in olive oil, lemon juice, pepper and salt to make a side salad.

Nutritional info: 197 calories, 12g fat, 1g net carbs, 21g protein

Day 5

Breakfast
Microwave-bread

Lunch
Previous night's dinner

Dinner

Slow cooker lemon garlic chicken

Day 6

Breakfast
Broccoli and Cheese Omelet

Lunch
Chicken salad with Basil-Lemon Vinaigrette

Dinner
Grilled Halloumi Salad

Day 7

Breakfast
Mini Frittata

Servings: 12

Ingredients

½ teaspoon salt

½ cup pepper jack cheese

10 eggs

1/3 cup liquid egg whites or 2 egg whites

¼ teaspoon pepper

8 ounces pork sausage

2 cups red & yellow diced sweet peppers

½ cup milk, 1%

Optional: fresh chopped cilantro, green onions, salsa, sour cream

Instructions

1. Preheat your oven to 350 degrees.

2. Heat a medium skillet and brown the sausage until it is cooked through.

3. Remove the sausage using a slotted spoon and set aside.

4. In the same skillet, add the peppers and sauté them until they are soft.

5. Whisk together the milk, eggs and egg whites in a large bowl.

6. Divide the peppers and sausage among a muffin tin (12-capacity tin). Pour the egg mixture evenly into each tin and sprinkle a generous tablespoon of cheese on top of each. Stir the mixture in each muffin cup using a fork.

7. Bake for about 25 to 30 minutes.

Nutritional info: 169 calories, 11.9g fat, 2.g net carbs, 11.2g protein

Lunch
Previous night's dinner

Dinner
Pecan crusted chicken

Conclusion

Thank you again for downloading this book!

I hope now you know that you can actually lose weight when you get started on a low carb diet. If getting started is a little bit challenging because you are used to high-carb foods, you can start by phasing out some high-carb foods like sodas, processed snacks and sugar. Once you get used, you can go a step further. Be patient and consistent and you will certainly lose weight and achieve your weight loss goals.

Finally, if you enjoyed this book, would you be kind enough to leave a review for this book on Amazon?

Thank you and good luck!

Made in the USA
Lexington, KY
25 March 2017